ENHANCE

BY NICK KOLTERMAN

YOUR PATH TO
HEALTHY, HAPPY FEET

Throne Publishing Group
2329 N Career Ave #215
Sioux Falls, SD 57107
ThronePG.com

ENHANCE

BY NICK KOLTERMAN

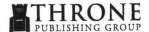

THRONE
PUBLISHING GROUP

"Nick has helped me with my foot problems for many years. This year we finally have conquered my ability to wear down a shoe in about 3 months. The new orthotics have held my feet in the correct position so I don't run over the sides of my shoes. This has been amazing and I am grateful for all his patience and willingness to work through this problem with me. Thank you Nick, for your kindness and patience."

Toni Hegna

"I've never learned so much about shoes until I came to Fit My Feet. I was having horrible pain in my feet when I worked out. I took my shoes into them and they showed me why I was having such pain and put me into a great pair of Brooks. Instantly, my foot pain was gone from my workouts. I would highly recommend going to Fit My Feet. You can't get this type of service at the box stores."

Carrie Bye Dragt

"I've been having issues for a year with metatarsalgia, and it just wasn't getting better. I decided to try this place to see if they could help and I am so thankful I did. Nick explained to me about the condition, gave some very helpful information, and let me know exactly what I needed to do. After I was fitted with a pair of very excellent Alegria shoes, the pain already improved. I was almost teary with relief and thankfulness. It was the most I have ever spent on footwear, but obviously I've been a little too cheap! This will be my shoe store from now on and I'm so grateful. Thank you Nick and Kathy - I'm a very satisfied customer!"

Lauri Hoffmann

"Nick Kolterman has a passion for teaching people how to care for their feet and helping those people who are suffering with problem/pain plagued feet. He was referred to me by my podiatrist. I not only needed his expertise in finding shoes that were compatible with my particular problems, but also required a custom molded splint for a toe that had been amputated. He was able to fit me with shoes that actually have the depth my feet require and is making the splint which I have needed for six years. My other foot was also causing me trouble due to an infected corn and callus. Nick checked it out, disappeared into his shop, and returned a few minutes later with a spacer-cushion designed by him. He also recommended socks which actually keep *my feet from sweating, control the growth of infection, and fit my swollen calves. Using the cushion and socks has solved my problem on this foot which had troubled me for a year. My shoes will be available this week as well as the material to be used to make the splint for my missing toe. As I have fallen several times in the past few years, I am very excited to finally find someone who understands and can help with foot problems.*

If you are reading this testimonial, then you have purchased or are considering purchasing his book: "Enhance: Your Path to Healthy, Happy Feet". Buy the book and learn from his training, experience, and expertise. Your feet will thank you!"

Rev. Raymon Sondergaard

"Nick and [the] staff are so helpful. They take the time to make sure you are comfortable and answer any questions you have. Love the staff!"

Denelle Wilson

"Where do you go when you have spent thousands of dollars on orthotics from three different professional pedorthists and no one can help you? I went to Nick Kolterman. He listened to me with interest and asked evaluative questions. His first counsel was to go buy a two-dollar toe separator that relieved a pinched nerve allowing me to walk again. From there he personally designed custom orthotics and selected specific shoes for my unique foot problems. The results speak for themselves. I ran a 5k the other day and thanked God for Nick, his servant leadership, and professional skills as a pedorthist."

Don LeClere

"I was so happy to find Nick at the Fit My Feet store. He originally got me going with the orthotic inserts he made for my shoes. Now I have happy feet wearing my fashionable Alegria clogs. Plus, I am actually wearing a pair of sneakers without the inserts. They are Altra Torins which are ultra lite and nicely cushioned. I am not a runner, but sure feel like I could run in these. Go see Nick if you have any foot problems---he is sure to get you moving again."

Tiffany Fay

"Over 10 years ago I walked into a local shoe store to buy another pair of tennis shoes like the ones I had. I guess it was my lucky day as Nick Kolterman was the one who came to wait on me. He took one look at my feet & said, "these aren't the shoes for you." At the time he was studying Pedorthics and Orthotic Fitter & working part time at the shoe store. He taught me more about my feet than anyone else I have been to in the past. I have multiple problems with my feet such as fallen arches, Tendonitis and Arthritis. Nick is very knowledgeable as to what to do to help the situation when it comes to foot pain. He has fit me with orthotics & as my feet have gotten progressively worse, he was able to tweak the ones I have to make my feet more comfortable. I wouldn't think of having anyone else fit my feet but Nick Kolterman."

Barb DeLange

"After searching for Nick after he left the Orthopedic Institute, we finally found him!! So grateful because myself, sister and nephew had gotten orthotics from him before and needed new ones and our old ones tweaked to feel better since they were broke down. He does a great job and is well worth it. We value his knowledge about our feet."

Karilyn Richards

"Two years ago I noticed my daughter was having trouble walking and playing sports. I was also struggling with plantar fasciitis and had been told by a co-worker that I should visit Nick at Fit My Feet. Nick was quick to pinpoint both of our troubles and what kind of shoes would help us. He made modifications to a pair of orthotics so that they worked specifically for my daughter's feet. Once getting the right shoes and inserts, everything corrected itself! We are grateful for Nick's expertise."

Kris Johnson

Acknowledgments

First and foremost I would like to thank Jesus Christ. Without him I would not be able to share my knowledge and expertise in helping people get better. I would like to thank my wife, Amanda for standing beside me throughout my career and writing this book. She has been my inspiration and motivation for continuing to improve my knowledge and move my career forward. She is my rock and always puts up with me and my crazy ideas as an entrepreneur. I would like to thank my parents for raising me in a Christian home and always believing in me and standing beside me in my career. I appreciate the knowledge, leadership, and love my parents; Paul and Charlene. To my kids, Caden and Kyleigh, who are the reason I get out of bed every morning to pursue my dreams.

I want to also thank the group of doctors I work with in the community. They put their trust in me to take care of their patients, and for that I say, "Thank You." I have learned a great deal from some of the physicians I have worked with over the years. To mention a few; Dr. Eric Watson, Dr. Brian Fay, Dr. Travis Venner, Dr. Adam Nichols, Dr. Jason Anderson, and Dr. Greg Neely.

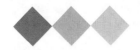

Table of Contents

1

Your Feet's Role in Holistic Health

Your Feet's Role in Holistic Health

Did you know that foot health is a vital aspect of your body's overall well-being? Everything starts from the ground up and your body is no exception. Your feet are your foundation: if you take care of them, they will take care of you. But, much like a house, if the foundation is not cared for problems will inevitably arise. This is why an attitude of prevention is crucial for a healthy body and feet.

One of my goals is to help folks solve problems before they even arise, and a simple method that's often overlooked is choosing the right pair of shoes and inserts. Shockingly, some people spend thousands of dollars on shoes only to realize that, after five or six pairs, they're still in the same pain. However, if you pick the right pair the first time you can save money and even months of discomfort. Better still is that having a proactive mindset when it comes to keeping your feet healthy can keep you upright and active far into the future.

> One of my goals is to help folks solve problems before they even arise.

It's no surprise, we're all living longer these days which means our feet will see more miles than ever. One simple secret to a high-quality of life as we age is taking care of issues while we're young—ideally, before they even happen! If you want your seventies and eighties to be active years, you're going to need healthy feet to make it happen. If you commit to taking care of your feet while you're young you can prevent a host of problems in the years ahead. Simply put, the healthier your feet, the happier your life.

You might think this is an exaggeration, but consider this: People constantly tell me that if their feet are hurting, they don't feel like doing anything. In fact, too many of my geriatric patients confide that they wish they had taken better care of their feet when they were younger. But the good news is that even something as simple as wearing the right shoes and quality inserts will help.

However, it's important to remember that foot health isn't simply a problem as you age. An attitude of preventing future pain is critical, but so is understanding the impact of foot health here and now. For instance, at birth many children have genetic issues such as congenital flatfoot. That condition is not their fault and isn't something that can be changed. So as parents, if you realize your daughter or son has foot pain, take care of it right away. Don't let it go. Even if a doctor tells you that the discomfort is simply due to growing pains, the underlying issue may be something more than that, something that we can help ease the pain. Let's face it, kids are more active these days.

Another great example is a woman we helped who went back to work after several years as a homemaker. Due to the nature of her new job, she was on her feet for eight to twelve hour stretches on concrete and tile floors. This is a case where proper shoe choice and inserts can bring tangible benefits today and set you up for healthy feet tomorrow. Unfortunately, many don't seek foot care until they're already experiencing a laundry list of issues. If you're experiencing dull, achy pains in the heel and ball of your foot, ankle instability, or any burning, tingling, and numbness in your toes, it's time to come see us to try a better shoe or your doctor.

> **Many don't seek foot care until they're already experiencing a laundry list of issues.**

However, when any of these symptoms arise, I encourage my patients to examine their feet. Do they hurt to the touch? Do they hurt when you run? When you walk? If you're active, be aware of your feet and pay attention to any onset of pain. Remember, your foot health impacts your overall wellness. So chances are, if you're experiencing problems in your feet, you will suffer adverse effects in your upper extremities as well.

This chain reaction happens because your feet are both kinetically and bio-mechanically connected to your ankles, knees, hips, and back. Think of it this way, the knee follows the foot and the hip follows the knee. Do you see how that works? This is why many ankle, knee, hip, and even back problems can arise from feet that are out of alignment. So when you're dealing with a foot problem or pathology, take care of it right away. Don't let it go! Otherwise you may end up with problems well beyond your feet.

At Fit My Feet, we try to prevent upper extremity issues through alignment by taking a holistic approach. We're not invasive, so we look at the kinetic and bio-mechanic elements of the foot. How far off is it? What type of foot do you have? How do we fix it? Then, when we have a diagnosis we can both prevent issues from worsening and alleviate pain, so you can enjoy life now and down the road. We don't want your pain to come back. Your feet are the first things to hit the ground. So, if they hurt you're not going to do certain things. For example, we have folks who come in and tell us they no longer run half-marathons or walk their dog in the morning because of foot pain.

Do you see what happens? People change their lifestyles based on foot pain. There are simply things many find themselves unable, or unwilling, to do when it hurts. Constant pain in your feet, knees, or back is miserable and can sap the fun out of activities that were once a joy. Now, there are a lot of things you can do to prevent or even get rid of that pain entirely. Unfortunately, many don't look for those answers and let the problem go until they've developed a chronic issue. Once that happens, they try to fight the problem, but often reach the wrong answers. For example, they may start taking pain medication instead of looking at the larger picture and making the necessary changes.

When it comes to your health, a great rule of thumb is that if discomfort is negatively impacting your lifestyle, it's time to see an expert. And remember, because your feet are kinetically attached to your ankles, knees, hips, and back, those joints may be achy because your feet are out of alignment. So whether it's through proper footwear or orthotics, we aim to support the foot the way it truly needs to be supported. And when we do this for your feet, they can properly support the rest of your body.

As humans, we try to adapt and compensate when we have problems. But the key is that we change the right things so that the real issues are solved rather than simply lived with. This is why seeking help and advice from experts is so important. The right diagnosis and subsequent treatment can be a real life changer.

Question 1

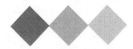

Where does your pain start and what makes the pain feel better?

Question 2

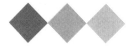

How long have you been dealing with the pain?

Question 3

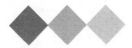

Does the pain come and go? Or is it a more chronic pain that has been around for a while?

2

Basic Foot Anatomy

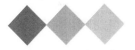

Basic Foot Anatomy

Just like our personalities, we all have different foot shapes. The three most common foot types are the normal arch, the high arch and the flat foot. Knowing what shape your feet are is important because your arch determines what shoe you need. Without that knowledge, finding the right shoes and inserts becomes very difficult. Which is why every time someone visits us at Fit My Feet, we identify your foot type and then, armed with this information, we can find the perfect shoe for you.

> The three most common foot types are the normal arch, the high arch and the flat foot.

The first and most common foot shape is the normal arch. It's simple and straightforward, just like it sounds. The arch is neither too high nor too low, it's normal. One great way to determine what kind of arch you have is to stand in front of a mirror and pay close attention to the angle of your ankles. They shouldn't be bent in or bowed out, but relatively straight up and down.

The second is the high arch, and is also known as a cavus foot. This means that the middle of your foot—the arch—may never touch the ground. If this sounds like your feet, one quick way to check is either by walking barefoot in the sand or standing on a tile floor with wet feet. If you can't see the middle of your foot in the footprints left on the sand or tile, that's a good indication that you may have a high arch.

Flat feet are the third type and happen to be the most common shape we see at Fit My Feet. This shape tends to cause the most problems later in life. And while there are a lucky few that suffer no problems at all, most flat footers will experience pathologies that develop with foot pain at some point. One of the most common ailments is plantar fasciitis—but more on that in a later chapter.

Arthritis

Finally, there are arthritic feet. Arthritis is a common foot problem and to best explain its impact on foot health, I have asked Dr. Brian Fay, MD, who is an excellent rheumatologist in the Sioux Falls area to contribute.

There are more than 100 types of arthritis (inflammation of 1 or more joints) that afflict persons of all ages. Osteoarthritis and rheumatoid arthritis are 2 common forms of arthritis that may affect the foot and ankle. Over 37% of all adults are affected by osteoarthritis (OA) with more joints being affected in women than men. Feet are commonly affected and symptoms can include pain, swelling, and localized joint pain.

Osteoarthritis (OA) is commonly known as "wear and tear" arthritis and represents the most common form of arthritis in the United States. It arises from degeneration of the cartilage with narrowing of the joint space and formation of bone spurs. This results in altered mechanics and increased stress on the joint and soft tissue structures (ligaments, tendons, and muscles) that support the joint. Common symptoms include stiffness, pain, and swelling which worsens with use of the affected joint(s). Osteoarthritis of the foot most commonly affects the base of the big toe and mid-foot. While there is no cure for osteoarthritis, many treatment options are available to improve comfort and slow the progression of disease.

Rheumatoid arthritis (RA) is a common autoimmune form of arthritis which predominantly affects the small joints of the hands and feet. In RA, the immune system mounts an inappropriate response against the lining of the joint (synovium) resulting in inflammation (synovitis). Left untreated, RA will destroy the joint, surrounding soft tissue structures, and underlying bone leading to pain, swelling, and deformities. RA is generally symmetrical and involves the ankle and joints at the base of the toes (metatarsophalangeal joints). In contrast to OA, RA symptoms worsen overnight and with inactivity. The goal of RA treatment is remission of disease and often requires multiple treatment modalities.

Dr. Fay explains that the medical management of arthritis involves pain medication, anti-inflammatory medication, physical therapy, proper fitting shoes, orthotics, and even braces.

Now, one of the most important reasons to know your foot shape is shoe choice. The shape of your foot determines the structure and support of your shoe. But, get this, no two feet in nature are the same—not even your own two feet! An interesting wrench nature likes to throw at us is that our own two feet may be different shapes. Sometimes one foot is longer. Other times one is wider. And in some rare cases we've seen folks with one flat foot and one high arch. That's an extreme difference in the same person. In fact, it's even possible to have a problem in one foot but not the other. Because there are so many variables when it comes to foot shape, getting expert help on shoe choice can alleviate a lot of pain down the road.

> **One of the most important reasons to know your foot shape is shoe choice.**

We see a lot of people with a foot shape that's caused an issue they've let go. So when someone comes in with a foot problem, one of the first things we want to know is how long they've dealt with it. And, often, in an issue caused by arch type, they've suffered for many years needlessly due to lack of education. People simply don't know that there are shoes and inserts designed specifically for their kind of foot that can alleviate pain.

This is especially true with high arches because, mechanically speaking, they are the most difficult arches to correct. They also cause the most lower extremity issues in the knees and the hips because high arches adversely affect the mechanical function of those joints. Remember, everything is kinetically attached and connected just like the children's song, "The knee bone's connected to the, leg bone…" It sounds simple, but it is easy to overlook. So, if an individual consults a doctor for knee pain, it might be the feet that are to blame. But this can be tricky to catch because the pain may actually be the symptom of a problem in another area—often the feet.

As practitioners, when we know what foot type you have, we can correctly identify and fix the source of your problems. This is important to understand because, in coming to us first, you may save significant time, money, and discomfort! Some folks go straight to the store and buy an over-the-counter product. But if they don't know their arch type, there is a good chance they might purchase the wrong product. For us, however, identifying your foot type is a top-priority because it's key in eliminating foot pain—and that's our job.

Recently, one of my podiatrist friends said to me, "If people treated their feet the way they treat their eyes, I'd be seeing a lot fewer patients." You know what? He's right. Think about it. If someone is going blind and can't see, they go to the doctor and drop $400 or $500 to get glasses or contacts. Of course, seeing is worth the price. But aren't your feet too?

Think about the warehouse worker on concrete all day or the cashier on hard tile. Those surfaces are tough on your feet, so getting the right support for your foot shape is absolutely worth the investment. And the time to make that investment is before the problems begin. We don't like to see people come in with severe pain they've lived with for months, or even years. They let it go and go until finally the pain has moved from their knees into their hips and they eventually can't walk. Pain spreads like wildfire because we involuntarily try to compensate for it by making unnatural adjustments in how we move another part of the body. What ends up happening is stress and strain on another area. Thus, the pain creeps from one joint to the next. Do yourself a favor and get ahead of discomfort by being properly fitted for shoes and inserts.

When you go into a department store and try on shoes or over-the-counter inserts, there may be times you won't know what you're buying. This has the propensity to cause more problems than it solves, because if you buy an insert made for high arches and you have a flat foot, you'll be in trouble. This is why it's important to know your feet and do your homework. When you do, you can make the educated choices necessary to make them feel better.

Another crucial element to foot health is having your feet measured. When you visit Fit My Feet we measure because it's important. The Brannock Device (the adjustable foot gadget that measures feet) was invented in the early 1900's for a good reason. Before the Brannock Device®, the available option was a primitive block of measured wood. The Brannock Device® dramatically improved the accuracy of a foot measurement, to 95-96 percent. The size system is linear. For example, a Men's size 1 is 7-2/3 inches. Each additional size is 1/3 inch longer. Widths work the same way. Each width is separated by a distance of 3/16 of an inch. There are actually nine widths in the

US system (width actually varies with foot length): AAA, AA, A, B, C, D, E, EE, and EEE.

The Brannock Device® comes in green, purple, red or black. There are models for men, women, athletic shoes, ski boots, and for children. The device has two knobs for adjusting the fit cups at both ends for the curve of the heel, and a sliding bar for adjusting "firmly for a thin foot, and lightly for a wide foot."

When we properly fit your foot shape with an accommodating shoe you will have fewer problems and less pain. Our job is to allow you to be on your feet all day without discomfort. We're here to make your feet happy.

But when you walk into an average shoe store you're surrounded by hundreds of options. There's a mammoth selection spanning all types and shapes. So how will you know which ones are the proper match for your feet? In a big-box store you generally try shoes on by yourself without the help of an expert to measure your feet and discern your foot shape and arch type. Sadly, you may walk away with a great looking pair of new shoes that will do murder to your feet. And where do shoes that hurt your feet end up? They go in the closet where they are no help to anyone.

Statistically, 78% of the population will develop a foot pathology of some sort. Wouldn't you like to know that you're being fitted for the right shoe? Would you like the chance to avoid being one of the 78-out-of-100? One of our biggest motivations in fitting people with the right shoes is pain prevention. We don't want you to hurt, and you certainly don't either!

Question 1

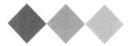

What type of arch do I have?
High, Medium or Flat?

Question 2

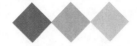

When was the last time I
had my feet measured?

Question 3

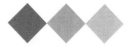

Do I have any foot deformities that need accommodative shoes?

3

How to Fit Your Feet

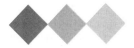

How to Fit Your Feet

Here's a scenario we see every day: a customer is experiencing foot pain and decides a new shoe can help alleviate it. So, they visit a big-box store and spend hours and better than a hundred dollars finding the shoe they think will do the job. Things are great, at first. But, guess what? Three or four months later they're having the same problems they were experiencing when they bought the new shoe.

The right shoe is instrumental in treating and preventing foot pain, but finding it can be a daunting, even frustrating, task. When you don't find the right fit, your problem is shifted down the line rather than resolved because the underlying issue remains untreated. So, an important question becomes, why does this happen and how can you avoid this situation?

How do I know I'm buying the right shoe?

The right shoe is determined by your foot shape and measurement. Even if a shoe feels good for a few moments in the store, it will ultimately fail to ease pain if it's not built for your foot type. When you walk into a shoe store, your number one concern should be your current foot measurements. And it's important to remember that they change over time.

A lot of folks are surprised to learn they don't wear the same sized shoe they did in high school. Our feet change as we age. For example, if you've gained some weight over the years, it will affect your feet. When you are heavier more force is exerted on your feet, which means they stretch out, getting wider and longer. This often happens to women during pregnancy as well. When they have children, their feet change. And, it is not unusual for feet size and shape to not return to their pre-pregnancy measurements due to pregnancy weight gain and swelling.

Because your feet change, getting accurate measurements before you buy is where the hunt for a new shoe must begin. When you visit a shoe store and the first thing they do is take your current measurements, it's a good sign that they know what they're doing. But, if they don't start there-run! If they don't know your measurements, the only way you're going to end up in the correct shoe is if you get lucky. It's just like winning the lottery. It's possible, but don't bet your future on it. At Fit My Feet we measure absolutely everyone's feet when they walk in the door. But measuring feet is about much more than knowing you wear a size nine-and-a-half.

Measuring Feet is About More Than Size

Your foot measurement is a combination of three variables: depth, width, and length. Your foot's depth is a measurement of how tall your foot is from the top to the sole. This helps us determine what height we need to look for in your new shoe. Width is the measurement of your foot at its widest point. However, this should be taken when you're standing as well as sitting, because when you put weight on your feet they splay and widen. Lastly, length is the figure most folks are familiar with; it's your foot's heel-to-toe measurement.

Your foot measurement is a combination of three variables: depth, width, and length.

Shoemakers understand these variables and make shoes to fit the many varieties of foot shapes and measurements. For instance, where the ball of your foot is located along the foot's length is very important because it lines up with the breaking point of the shoe. Factors and details like these contribute to the way each brand and model of shoe is made. This is great news, because it means there's always a shoe for you. The trick is finding it.

Now what makes the right shoe? It's pretty simple. The perfect fit is the one that corrects your problem and feels great the moment you hit the sidewalk. This means the notion of a "break-in period" is dead wrong. Your new shoe should feel good and correct your problem within the first couple weeks. Often, when a shoe is too tight beneath the laces people think (or are told) that it will stretch and fit better once it's worn for a while. But if it's the right fit, there shouldn't be any break-in time at all. The proper shoe relieves pain and perfectly complements your foot from your steps. Once you're in the right shoe, there are three primary benefits you can expect from the get go.

Three Benefits of Having the Right Shoe

The right shoe is the one that fits well, feels good, and lasts a long time. There won't be any slippage in the heel. There won't be blisters or uncomfortable tightness beneath the laces. Your pain will disappear. It will support you well in your chosen activities, and it will have maximum longevity. After all, what's the point of finding the perfect shoe if you can't enjoy it for a long time? It needs to stand up to what you intend to use it for.

When you find the right shoe, these three benefits will be there every time. However, because everyone's feet are unique, there are no absolutes when treating foot pathologies and pain. Because feet are structurally different, the $150 shoe that corrected your friend's plantar fasciitis may not help yours. What works well in one situation may not work in another. This means that, even with the same diagnosis, individuals may still need radically different treatments.

Shoes are never a one-size-fits-all affair because people have different gaits, foot shapes, measurements, and weights. This is why it's vitally important that the folks you buy your shoes from understand that your foot is unique. Your path to the shoe that fits well, feels good, and lasts a long time will be dependent on what is unique about you. At Fit My Feet our job is to help you find that perfect shoe.

How Do We Find the Right Shoe?

Now that we know having the right shoe is crucial to alleviating pain, treating pathologies, and finding greater enjoyment in an active lifestyle, you're probably wondering *how* we do it. By now this shouldn't come as a surprise, but we begin the process by measuring, measuring, measuring! Your measurements dictate which shoes and manufacturers we'll explore with you for several reasons. And here's where an interesting facet of our expertise comes into play.

When shoes are made they're built around something called a shoe last. It is essentially a proxy that acts as a fake foot for the makers to craft shoes around. The lasts are contoured to mimic a wide variety of foot shapes and measurements, and shoemakers have them for every half-size, full-size, and width. It's important for your shoe experts to be well-acquainted with this process because this is where everything starts. Even before shoes hit the shelves they're made for a specific foot shape. For every shape there's a shoe. And there's a last for every foot shape!

Shoes are a combination of many parts brought together to support unique foot shapes. And we need to know our shoe anatomy to best decide which components will compliment your feet and their intended activities. This is where the experts come in. However, at Fit My Feet, we also think it's important to listen and observe.

Sometimes professionals assume they know everything. But often they don't listen for helpful clues because they've already made assumptions or generalized a customer's needs. Rather than assuming, we listen for key pieces of information. Did your last pair of shoes fit properly? Were your boots too tight in the toe box? Are there areas where you have pain? Where are they? Do you need a wider or longer shoe this time? When we listen, we already know what we're *not* going to put you in, and that's half the battle. We eliminate certain shoes when we realize they won't fit your needs.

In addition to listening and making observations, we ask questions. What is your desired outcome for the new shoe? Is it a business shoe or will you be running marathons in it? If it's for work, are you in an office or are you a waitress and need a non-slip shoe? Are you a farmer who needs durability and protection? Are you a retail worker on hard, tile floors all day? When we better understand how you're going to use the shoe, we're even closer to the perfect pair.

Another major consideration is whether or not you need orthotics. A key component of what we do as practitioners is fitting inserts. Whether it's an over-the-counter orthotic or one we've custom made, we do this everyday to help take the pain away. And what's interesting is that the shoe we'd put you in with an insert is not the same one we'd put you in without one.

The dynamics of an insert change the shoe fit. It also changes your gait. Often people want to be kept in the same shoe even when adding an orthotic, but this is frequently not the best fit. It's our job to know that and help you understand why. If we've built an insert for the wrong shoe then it's not going to help. Similarly, if we put you in the right shoe with the wrong orthotic we're not getting anywhere either. The two have to mesh together to accomplish our primary goal: correct the problem to take the pain away.

We consider how the orthotic and shoe will work together because we don't want to overcorrect your foot. If they don't complement each other they'll do more harm than good. An overcorrected foot isn't much, if any, better than an untreated one. Thus, when you go to Walmart and step onto the Dr. Scholl's pad and it spits out an orthotic number, nine-times-out-of-ten you'll be no better off because the insert isn't paired with the proper shoe. The wrong insert negatively changes the mechanics of a shoe. This is why you come to the experts, because we give you direction on fit *and* function in the interplay between shoes and orthotics.

Our Work Isn't Done Yet!

At Fit My Feet, if we know your foot measurements, ask the right questions, and then listen, we'll get you into the right shoe every time. But, guess what? Even after we've found the perfect pair for you, our work isn't done! Our expertise stretches beyond shoe and orthotic selection. For us, it's details time. There are two areas we like to focus on once we've gotten you into the right shoe: lacing technique and shoe modification.

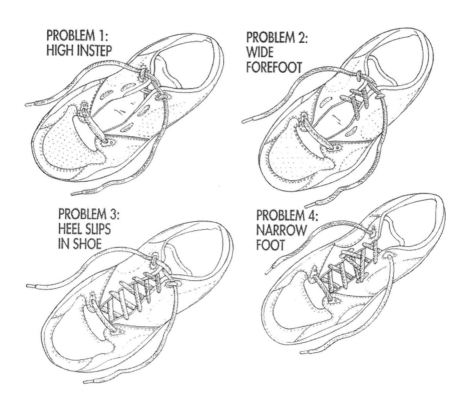

PROBLEM 1:
HIGH INSTEP

PROBLEM 2:
WIDE
FOREFOOT

PROBLEM 3:
HEEL SLIPS
IN SHOE

PROBLEM 4:
NARROW
FOOT

Lacing technique is a lost art that goes above and beyond fitting. Many don't know this, but there are several ways to lace a shoe. Knowing which shoe lacing method to use can help you relieve that last little bit of foot pain. Are you a runner and getting some heel slippage? Do you have bunions, bony prominences, or arthritis? These are all problems we can address with one of three lacing techniques: the skip lace, the runner's lace (also called the loop lace), and the stop lace.

The skip lace is primarily used to relieve pain on the top of arthritic feet. With this technique we're skipping certain laces to avoid pain and bony prominences in the foot. Then we get creative with your lacing pattern, which even more closely tailors your shoes to your feet.

The runner's lace helps to stop heel slippage and micro-motion in the shoe. You may have never noticed, but every pair of running shoes has an extra eyelet at the back of the shoe. This has been around for decades yet few people take advantage of it. It is used to alleviate achilles tendon pain, heel pain, blisters, and micro-motion. All of these issues can be avoided by lacing the shoe just a bit differently to control those painful variables.

Finally, the stop lace is a great all-around technique. It adds more function and helps the shoe hug the foot more closely. Again, this reduces abrasive rubbing, slippage, and micro-motion that cause discomfort and pain.

So far, we've found the wearer's fit and determined lacing. What could be left? The final consideration is whether or not your new shoe could benefit from modification. We modify shoes in several ways and determine which of the many techniques at our disposal to use. For instance, does the patient or consumer have a bunion? Do they have a problem with the toe line? Do they have a hammer toe? We have an industrial shoe stretcher to address these very issues.

For example, some folks have a bunion so painful that it's forced them to buy shoes three sizes wider to accommodate it. However, this ultimately resulted in a shoe that didn't fit well everywhere else and caused more problems than it solved. We can avoid this misfitting by strategically stretching the new shoe to account for a unique need.

Another simple, yet effective, modification we make is tongue pads. A frequent cause of heel slippage is having the wrong tongue pad. So we simply change to one that takes pressure off of the top of the foot to reduce the slippage and provide a snugger fit at the instep.

There are so many solutions to every problem; you simply need a professional shoe provider who can help you find the right one. We can make those final adjustments to get your shoe fitting just the way you need it. Our goal is to find a shoe that fits well, feels good, and lasts you

> Our goal is to find a shoe that fits well, feels good, and lasts you a long time.

a long time. So we measure, listen, ask questions, make orthotics, and expertly leverage every option available to us to get you into the perfect shoe. This is how we fit your feet.

Question 1

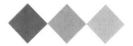

What brand of shoe do you currently wear and why?

Question 2

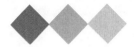

What size have I been wearing in that shoe?
What width do I fit into the best?

Question 3

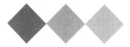

Do I lace my shoes to relieve pressure from the foot?
Is there any abnormal wear on the soles of my current shoes?

4

How to Prevent Future Foot Problems

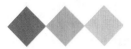

How to Prevent Future Foot Problems

We treat a diverse range of foot pathologies each year. From misaligned feet and ankles to diabetes with accompanying foot disease, we see it all. However, there are four pathologies we see more than any others: plantar fasciitis, achilles tendonitis, metatarsalgia, and medial tibial stress syndrome (also known as shin splints).

Though each is unique and requires a nuanced approach, there is a common thread in how we treat them all. Our constant goal is to relieve pain and prevent it in the future, which means our job is to fit you with the perfect shoe and orthotic. These four problems, while painful, are each treatable and preventable. So, if you presently struggle with one of them, or even think you might be, then do yourself a favor and pay us a visit!

When I talk with patients suffering from a pathology, I explain that there are three stages to any problem. There's the initial stage in which an individual has mild pain. They may be experiencing a dull ache in the heel or occasional discomfort in the ball of the foot. It hurts, but it's not keeping the individual from regular activity. The second stage is typified by acute pain. At this point things have progressed from irregular and minor discomfort to sharp pains and persistent aches. The patient may begin to experience trouble walking normal distances and the pain makes activity unpleasant. And lastly, the third stage is where folks experience chronic pain. These individuals are dealing with significant pain for months. The pain is persistent and the problem intensifies over time.

Unfortunately, too many people wait to come and see us until they've reached the second or third stage. They visit only after the pain has negatively impacted their quality of life. So, as we look at these four common pathologies, remember that foot pain doesn't have to be a way of life. Come in and let us help you on your way to pain free feet.

Plantar Fasciitis

As pedorthists, plantar fasciitis is the most common diagnosis we treat. The plantar fascia is the thick connective tissue that supports the longitudinal arch in the foot. It runs from the heel bone to the metatarsal (ball of the foot) and functions much like a tendon. When a patient suffers from plantar fasciitis, he or she experiences pain in the heel caused by stress or micro-tears in their underfoot tissue.

Remember that foot pain doesn't have to be a way of life.

Folks with plantar fasciitis will usually notice pain in the morning when their feet first hit the floor. Sufferers experience achiness when standing or walking on tile, hardwood floors, and other firm surfaces. The pain will typically be localized at the base of the heel. It often presents in dull, achy pains or as sharp pain sporadically throughout the day. Heel spurs can also develop alongside plantar fasciitis, which can cause micro-tears in the plantar fascia if the spur is not offloaded in the heel.

Though this ailment can happen to anyone, we most frequently treat it in athletes with high arches. This occurs when their connective tissue, the plantar fascia, is inflexible. After all, what happens to rigid connectors under stress? They pull and tear. Athletes put significant load on their feet. They're constantly sprinting, jumping, cutting, and training which puts tremendous pressure on the plantar fascia.

However, the pain isn't simply limited to athletes. We also see it in people with poor fitting shoes and those with flat feet as well as those with high arches. Poor fitting shoes are a perpetual problem because they offer inadequate support to the arch. Additionally, people with flat feet experience pain because their arch elongates too far. So, as the foot stretches and the arch drops, the plantar fascia is stretched and stressed too far; causing pain, inflammation, and possibly tearing.

Generally, people who come to us with plantar fasciitis have been diagnosed by a podiatrist and written prescriptions for well-fitting shoes and custom orthotics. Then a pedorthist will treat based upon the diagnosis we're dealing with. Our goal is to treat the pathology non-invasively. We don't like to see our patients go to the surgery room—and most doctors agree with us on that! Good doctors don't like to cut unless they have to.

> **Poor fitting shoes are a perpetual problem because they offer inadequate support to the arch.**

When we're treating plantar fasciitis non-invasively we begin by alleviating stress on the tissue. Sometimes we need to decrease pronation (the rolling over of the foot) because it causes stress to the connective tissue. We also modify shoes, fabricate orthotics and ensure we have the arches properly supported. It often takes a combination of all of these things to alleviate tension on the plantar fascia. However, there are occasions when a non-invasive cure is not possible. When necessary, a podiatrist will perform a fasciotomy, which is a surgical procedure where the fascia is cut to reduce the problematic tension.

While plantar fasciitis is common, it can also be serious if left untreated. For instance, one patient I treated was forced to go on disability because the pain had all but crippled him. It sounds crazy, but it's true. We've also treated many patients who've changed jobs because their foot pain was too severe to continue in a career that kept them on their feet all day.

Chronic pain changes the way we live—and always for the worse. Whether it's plantar fasciitis or another pathology, when you're forced to change jobs or cut back on activities because of foot pain, it's time to start doing something differently. Often, this begins with well-fitting shoes and orthotics.

Achilles Tendonitis

Whenever you see a word with the suffix -itis, think inflammation. In this case, achilles tendonitis is the inflammation of the achilles tendon, which connects the heel with the calf muscles in your lower leg. The pain and swelling are caused by overuse. This tendon plays a mechanical role in our forward motion. Thus, runners, basketball players, tennis players, or anyone else who puts high strain on their achilles are susceptible to this injury—especially when the tendon is tight.

Those with achilles tendinitis typically notice pain at the insertion of the tendon in the heel, though it can travel up into the lower leg. This pain will often be accompanied by redness, puffiness, and increased pain at the back of the foot. Even if the symptoms seem mild, it's important to make sure you're fitted in the right shoe to avoid a rupture or a tear—which can sideline an athlete for months.

To treat the injury and relieve the symptoms, we need to first alleviate pressure on the achilles. This means we don't want you in a shoe that presses directly on the tendon in the back of the foot. However, if the issue is the heel bone itself, then the problem is caused by excessive torque placed on the tendon. In fact, when the achilles is out of alignment, the torque that's placed both on it, and the heel, is equal to three to four times an individual's body weight. When under that great of force, the tendon will typically become inflamed.

When we use orthotics to treat achilles tendonitis, we place them to realign the heel bone, and thus relieve stress from the tendon. Fortunately, we can do this even if you have a high arch or a flat foot. If, however, the tendon is extremely tight, we'll use a heel-lift in either the shoe's heel or in the orthotic we're making. This typically raises the heel by one-eighth of an inch. The lift reduces tension on the tendon because it no longer needs to stretch as far. The tendon is very similar to a rubber band. If a rubber band is stretched wide between our hands, it will be tight. But, if we bring the ends closer together the strain is reduced. It is the same with the achilles tendon. If we can use an orthotic to move the bottom end of the tendon closer to the top, strain is reduced. Most of the time the heel lifts are short-term and only need to be worn for six to eight weeks, or until the tendon settles down.

Metatarsalgia

A third common pathology we treat is metatarsalgia, which is pain and inflammation that occurs in the metatarsal (ball of the foot). Essentially, it's a layman's term for patients who present complications in a single metatarsal or all of the phalangeal joints. With metatarsalgia, the pain is greater with weight bearing and can cause callus formation as well. Sufferers often describe it as feeling like a stone is in their shoe or a wadded up sock is stuffed beneath the ball of their foot.

If you're experiencing a dull, achy pain in the balls of your feet, one thing you can do is self-examine. Simply look at the bottoms of your feet and note if there is any callusing. Is there a callus beneath the metatarsal where you are experiencing pain? If so, come in and see us! We can insert a metatarsal pad or bar to release tension from the ball of the foot.

While anyone may be inflicted with metatarsalgia, this pathology is also common to athletes. If, upon self-examination, you think you may have metatarsalgia, it's best to begin with your doctor and get a proper diagnosis. We want to know exactly what's going on so we can find the quickest path between you and pain-free feet. Unfortunately, when some people try to self-treat, they'll go to the store and buy four or five Dr. Scholl's pads and layer them in their shoes for extra padding. While padding is a key in relieving metatarsalgia pain, it's only half the battle. What they're failing to do is achieve proper alignment in the foot from a well-fit custom orthotic or pad. Ultimately, they're not treating the problem at all, only one of the symptoms.

When we treat metatarsalgia, we focus on softer soled shoes and inserts, but we ensure they're properly fit to your foot shape. It's also important for us to consider what kind of surfaces our patients will spend time on. For instance, a soccer player on grass is not likely to experience as much pain as a runner on pavement. Once we've discovered what surfaces the patient spends time on and find the proper fit, we select the appropriate shoe that's softer and more shock absorbent in the ball of the foot.

Additionally, we can fit people with a supportive metatarsal pad or bar, which reduces stress on the ball of the foot. Sometimes this is the best method of pain mitigation. We can also opt to use donuts or a custom made or fit orthotic. Whatever the solution, relieving tension for the phalangeal joints is the name of the game when treating metatarsalgia.

Medial Tibial Stress Syndrome

Medial tibial stress syndrome, commonly known as shin splints, is pain experienced along the medial region of the shin bones. It's generally the result of hyperpronation. Abnormal pronation places significant pressure on the tendon, which holds the muscle to the bone and results in excessive stress on its fibers. Again, it is similar to the rubber band analogy. When the foot is not in alignment with the leg, excessive tension is placed on the tendon resulting in pain. It's a chain reaction caused by misalignment. The process of tendon fibers being torn from the bone results in shin splints.

However, the foot does not necessarily have to hyperpronate for shin splints to occur. Sometimes we see someone with a high arch whose foot pronates to the outside of the foot from heel strike to toe off. This can result in shin splints as well. But, whatever the pronation, we need to correct the underlying musculoskeletal issue to bring the foot and leg into realignment. We need to relieve pressure on the tendon to take the pain away.

Our goal is to ensure that folks leave our office pain-free and do not return for the same issue. We want our clients to continue into health because we've promptly taken care of their alignment needs. However, just like yearly eye exams and physicals, make regular foot measurements a routine to ensure your feet are properly fit in the future. For as they say, "An ounce of prevention is worth a pound of cure."

Question 1

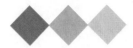

Am I experiencing pain? Where? If so, is there any swelling or redness where the pain is?

Question 2

Does it hurt to the touch?

Question 3

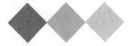

Does the pain remain consistent throughout the day or are there specific times of the day the pain increases?

5

Diabetes Impact on Foot Health

Diabetes Impact on Foot Health

Our feet are a gateway to optimum health. Pain-free feet support an active lifestyle and mobilize well-being. But, as we've explored in previous chapters, feet that hurt hamper us in nearly every facet of life. Sometimes we experience injuries. Other times ill-fitting shoes or orthotics are the culprits of discomfort. However, did you know that one-in-ten people are at risk of severe foot pathologies regardless of injury or improper footwear?

> **Pain-free feet support an active lifestyle and mobilize well-being.**

Over 29 million Americans have diabetes, a disease that can result in dangerously high blood sugar levels. Not only is diabetes a threat to a sufferer's heart, nervous system, and kidneys—it's also a liability to foot health. Diabetes can result in poor blood flow and loss of feeling (called neuropathy) in a patient's feet and legs. This has serious health implications, such as ulcers and infection, which can make amputation of the limb necessary. The good news is that if you suffer from diabetes, it doesn't have to spell doom for your feet! There are several ways that we help patients treat diabetes related foot ailments and aid in preventing common risk factors. But better health always starts with an understanding of both the problem and quality treatment.

How Can Diabetes Affect My Foot Health?

With such a significant portion of the US affected, it's important that we understand the real threat this disease poses to us through our feet. When someone lives with diabetes, proper foot care can be one of the first lines of defense against further serious complications. This is a facet of treatment that can even be overlooked by doctors who regularly see diabetic patients. Folks are prescribed medicine, undergo blood tests and lab workups, but the feet can be forgotten.

While the statistics concerning diabetes and related foot problems are shocking, understanding them is vital to helping combat harm to tens of thousands. Remember, one-out-of-every-ten people you see at work, in the grocery store, and even your family reunions, lives with diabetes every day. Since 1990, the disease has increased by a staggering 49% and is now the sixth leading cause of death in the United States. But how does diabetes pose a risk to our feet?

As discussed in the last chapter, infections are a serious threat to our overall health, and in diabetic patients, the feet are a common host of these infections. One of the disease's primary effects is neuropathy. Neuropathy is a type of nerve damage that results in pain, tingling, and numbness in the feet and extremities. These symptoms are mild for some, but for many others diabetic neuropathy can result in severe pain, immobilization, amputation, and even death.

For example, here's a situation we see often: a grandparent suffers from diabetes and has lost feeling in his or her lower extremities. One evening grandpa or grandma steps on a Lego resulting in a cut, but due to the numbness in the foot, cuts, wounds, and sores go unnoticed. Even if they're small, untreated cuts and scrapes pose a risk of infection. Unfortunately, since the individual doesn't feel the pain, he or she continues with normal day-to-day activities. Meanwhile, the cut worsens and becomes infected. Now, in the absence of pain, how can the patient discover the infected site? Blood. The wound often goes unnoticed until it, or effects of it, are seen. By then a serious problem has possibly developed because infected sores and open wounds can lead to foot or even leg amputation.

Another frequent scenario is related to poor footwear. We see a lot of diabetic folks walking around in a $29.99 K-Mart special shoe. Wearing an improper fitting shoe puts an individual at greater risk of getting ulcers, which can lead to infection, and ultimately the loss of a leg. Foot care becomes extremely important in diabetic patients because of their feet's susceptibility to wounds. In fact, 14-24% of diabetic patients have ulcers, appearing as a hole in the foot, caused by misfit shoes. This means they're in a shoe that is the wrong length, width, or depth for their foot shape. Proper footwear is one of the quickest paths to preventing such issues.

The leading cause of non-traumatic lower extremity amputations in the United States is diabetes. Approximately 14-24% of diabetics who develop foot ulcers will require an amputation (American Podiatric Medical Association). This year 82,000 diabetics will have a foot or leg amputated, and over $1 billion will be spent on those procedures. As practitioners, we do everything we can to prevent this because a sobering 39-68% of all leg amputees pass away within five years. That's a devastatingly high mortality rate.

So What Can I Do?

The first thing you can do, upon diagnosis from a medical professional, to get ahead of diabetes related problems in your feet is visit us at Fit My Feet. If you have already been diagnosed with diabetes, don't delay, come in today. This disease is something you may deal with for the rest of your life, but, if you take

> **Diabetes, left untreated in the feet, leaves you far more susceptible to developing attendant problems.**

preventative measures, you can avoid many of the negative consequences we've discussed. While there are some diabetics that don't end up with ulcers, infections, or neuropathy, don't count on being one of them. The math is not in your favor. Diabetes, left untreated in the feet, leaves you far more susceptible to developing attendant problems.

Understand that because of poor circulation in the feet, you may lose sensation and put yourself at a greater risk for ulcers and infections. But being fit in the right shoes and orthotics goes a long way in prevention. For example, one of the risks proper shoes and inserts can help prevent is called pre-ulcerated callousing. What happens is that folks who've lost much, or all sensation in their feet, can develop callouses on the bottoms of their feet from improper footwear. These callouses can then turn into underfoot ulcers, which again places you at a significantly higher risk for infection and eventually amputation.

A suggestion we make, in addition to wearing the correct shoe and insert, is a daily foot examination. Just take a look at your feet. Do you notice callouses or cuts? Do you see scrapes developing, or redness around the edges? Are there any open wounds or ulcers? Even minor abrasions can pose a health risk, so any of these should be immediately treated to prevent infection. We know some may have physical difficulties in conducting an examination. If this is the case, use a mirror to self-examine. Simply put your feet up to it and check the bottoms, sides, and any other places you're unable to see.

Our goal is keeping you healthy and moving.

Diabetes is an increasingly prevalent problem in our society, and the list of patients affected is increasing annually. However, if you or someone you know is diagnosed, please remember that foot health is paramount in preventing further complications, and know that we can help! You have options and can receive expert advice and care at Fit My Feet. Our goal is keeping you healthy and moving.

Your Do's & Don'ts for Diabetic Feet

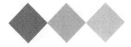

Do:

Inspect your feet daily for any signs of blisters, scratches, cuts, or sores. Always check between the toes.

Wear shoes that are made to protect your feet and do not leave them exposed.

If your feet feel cold, always wear socks to bed and in your shoes.

Regularly inspect the inside of your shoes for any foreign objects.

Visit your physician regularly and be sure to have them do a foot exam.

Your Do's & Don'ts for Diabetic Feet

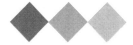

Don't:

Don't walk barefoot.

Don't use oils or creams between your toes unless prescribed by your doctor.

Don't cut corns or callouses by yourself.

Don't wear shoes with pointed toe areas or that create pressure.

6

Diabetic Feet Education

Diabetic Feet Education

Diabetes is a top-ten cause of death in the United States and poses a serious threat to our health and well-being. In the last chapter we looked at foot-related risk factors all diabetics face, from ulcers and infection to neuropathy and amputations, the potential consequences are severe. And, with such a high number of people affected, many wonder what diabetes is and who is at risk.

What is Diabetes Mellitus?

Diabetes Mellitus is a serious chronic metabolic condition resulting in high blood glucose levels. High glucose results from a deficiency in insulin, which is essential in the process of converting sugar into the energy our cells require. If left untreated, diabetes can result in blindness, kidney failure, stroke, or even amputation due to poor circulation in the lower extremities.

There are two types of diabetes: type one and type two. Type one diabetics are often called "insulin dependent," because most sufferers rely on daily insulin shots. This type is generally a juvenile or young adult onset—though it occurs later in rare instances. Type two diabetics are referred to as "non-insulin dependent," because most don't rely on insulin to control blood glucose levels. This type of diabetes will typically set in as an adult, often

> # Diabetes Milletus is a serious chronic metabolic condition resulting in high blood glucose levels.

developing in those in their thirties and forties. Most often, type two occurs in aging individuals who are overweight and live a sedentary lifestyle.

The most common diabetic complication is called, "foot disease with diabetes," and results in a 15% higher chance of developing foot ulcers with neuropathy. This diagnosis is objectively determined by lab tests that check for sensation in the feet, look for skin alteration indicative of poor circulation, and assess foot deformities. Diabetic effects may also coincide with different medical conditions such as human growth hormone supplementation, Cushing's disease, and peripheral vascular disease.

Peripheral vascular disease is caused by poor blood circulation and reduces oxygen and nutrients to tissues, worsens skin integrity, and puts the foot at significant risk. Poor circulation also impairs healing processes. Thus, if you have a wound or an ulcer, it won't heal as fast. This greatly increases a diabetics risk for infection and possible amputation. Well-fitting shoes and inserts speed up the healing process and lower amputation risk. So, clearly, the right fit is crucial for every diabetic.

What Products Can Help?

Diabetics today have more quality footwear options than ever before, and getting into the right products makes a world of difference. There are several quality lines of diabetic shoes and custom orthotics designed for patients with co-existing foot disease, but what's the difference between a specialty diabetic shoe and one from a department store?

Diabetics today have more quality footwear options than ever before, and getting into the right products makes a world of difference.

First, diabetic shoes undergo a rigorous testing process by shoe companies to meet Medicare and health insurance guidelines. In order to receive official approval as a diabetic shoe, it must be designed and constructed with significant differences in the toe box, vamps, and other key areas. Just like any other shoe, a diabetic shoe's design process begins with a last—the foot-mimicking mold that the shoe is built around, but these lasts differ because they imitate the specific needs of diabetic feet. Diabetic shoes typically have greater depth in the toe box (the front of the shoe where the toes splay), three width options for each length size (normal, wide, and extra-wide), flexibility in the vamp (top of the shoe), and adjustability in the lacing.

Ample depth in the toe box is critical for diabetic patients because it ensures there is no additional pressure placed on the tops of the toes. This goes a long way in aiding other pathologies as well. For example, if you're a diabetic with a hammertoe, rubbing will cause significant discomfort and pain. The toe box in a diabetic shoe is designed to remove friction and pressure.

Stretchy vamps are another crucial component in a diabetic shoe. The vamps stretch to fit the foot and accommodate pitting edema or significant swelling. A stretchy vamp's purpose is to expand and contract with the foot. When the foot is swollen, the vamp needs to give, but when swelling is reduced, it needs to follow the foot back to its normal size. Without a stretchy vamp, a diabetic's shoe can alternate from painfully tight to clunky and loose. For this reason, diabetic patients should avoid all-leather shoes, as they won't expand and allow the foot room with swelling. This can cause significant pain and discomfort.

Another important facet of a diabetic shoe is adjustability in the lacing. In fact, most slip-ons won't work for diabetic patients because they are rigid and unforgiving. That's why at Fit My Feet, we'll often put them in a shoe with laces or Velcro. We also see geriatric patients with mobility limitations or arthritis in addition to their diabetes. For these cases we like shoes with a one or two closure diabetic straps. This allows for easy maintenance and affords needed flexibility.

One of our primary goals is to alleviate pressure, and therefore pain, in swollen feet. A common source of this pain is in the stitching that digs into the top or sides of the foot. This is why we like seamless shoes for diabetics, which have no stitching in the toe to prevent rubbing, friction, and pressure. A major concern for diabetics is pre-ulcerated callusing that leads to an ulcer, sore, or wound that results in a hospital stay. Seamless shoes can go a long way in preventing these complications. For diabetics, it's especially important to get into the right shoe because it increases both long-term health and immediate comfort.

Quality Brands

Shopping for the right shoe can feel overwhelming, and it becomes even more so when you couple it with an additional diabetic need. With hundreds of options in most big-box stores, how can you know which shoe will help take the pain away and prevent future problems? For starters, if you're diabetic you simply must get fit in a diabetic shoe. Your feet have needs above and beyond what most non-diabetic shoes are designed to fulfill, so always begin your search by finding shoes built specifically for diabetic feet.

There are also several high-quality brands of diabetic shoe. For example, New-Balance is a fantastic company when it comes to diabetic shoes. You can buy their shoes almost anywhere and they offer a wide-range of options. However, they make both a low-end and a high-end diabetic shoe, so being educated on the difference between them and the potential impact to your health is critical. We trust several other brands as well: Orthofeet, Aravon (especially great for women), Dr. Comfort, and Aetrex Shoes. Not only can you buy everyday diabetic shoes from these brands, but some of them even make steel-toe diabetic work boots and slip-resistant diabetic work shoes. This means that no matter your needs and occupation, there's a shoe for you.

Diabetic Orthotics

Just like diabetic shoes, diabetic orthotics must be made specifically to suit a patient's needs. This means they'll be different than a sports or standard orthotic because they need the right balance of cushion and support. Also, they must be made with special materials that lessen the friction between the feet, socks, and shoes. This helps prevent additional pressure that can lead to calluses. In addition to orthotics, we use sheer pads to prevent pre-ulcerated callusing and ulcers.

Prevention

If you're diabetic, please don't wait until you have a problem to come in and see us. Let us help you get ahead of the pain! A proper fit is paramount in preventing ulcers, foot pain, and the host of other problems we've discussed. A preventative approach will keep you healthier, happier, more mobile, and better able to live with diabetes.

Question 1

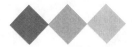

Have I visited with my doctor about diabetic shoes and orthotics?
Have I replaced my diabetic shoes and orthotics within the past year?

Question 2

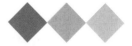

Do I have hammer toes or bunions that need to be accommodated by a better shoe for my diabetes?

Question 3

Do I check my feet on a daily basis?

7

Gaining an Athletic Edge

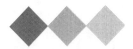

Gaining an Athletic Edge

Every year, thousands of athletes take to the track, field, and court. Each wants to be the quickest, sharpest, and strongest, so they train hard. They spend long hours before and after classes, at nights, and on weekends conditioning to gain that fourth-quarter advantage. Every athlete, no matter their age, wants an edge.

On top of training, thousands of dollars are spent on the right pads and equipment to play their game. Tennis players need rackets. Golfers need clubs. Baseball players need bats. Every sport requires a unique set of tools to be played, but there is one universal need every athlete, but a swimmer, has: shoes.

The right footwear and orthotics give athletes an edge. The right fit supports them as they cut, sprint, and jump. The perfect orthotic can even add the stability necessary to shave those last few seconds from a race time. But most of all, proper shoes and orthotics prevent the injuries that sideline hard working athletes every year. For a competitor, few things are worse than training day-in and day-out only to be sidelined with an injury on game day; especially when some of the most common injuries can be prevented.

At Fit My Feet there are four main injuries we see every season: achilles tendonitis, metatarsalgia, patella femoral syndrome, and posterior tibial stress syndrome. Though each affects a different area, they're all treatable and preventable through proper footwear. Each sport has unique demands and movements, and with ill-fitting shoes or inserts, problems arise in the form of pain and decreased performance.

Achilles Tendonitis

The achilles is the tendon that stretches from the heel to a muscle called the soleus, which is just below the calf on the back of the leg. Achilles tendonitis is a condition where this tendon has become inflamed. The achilles plays a key role in propelling us forward and is constantly at work as we walk and run. It can become inflamed in a number of ways, but the three most frequent causes are overuse, external factors, and flat-footedness. The external factors often include improper footwear and too much stress on the tendon when fully stretched.

One of the easiest treatments (and preventions) is to select and wear proper shoes and inserts—and this has been a theme throughout the book because I can't stress enough how important it is. For instance, we can modify a patient's shoes to make a gap at the back of the shoe, on the top of the heel to reduce stress on the tendon, or we can place wedges in the heel or build custom orthotics to alleviate stress, tension, and pain. Additionally, we work one-on-one with physical therapists to fix the condition biomechanically. Our goal is to address the problem with the athlete's motion through the plane of the heel and relieve tension in the tendon.

On top of ill-fitting footwear and harmful motion, an athlete's foot shape can be the root of the problem. A flat foot can result in too much torque on the tendon which produces amplified stress. When this happens, the foot cannot shock absorb well, and in turn, the weight exerted on the tendon is equal to up to four-times the individual's body weight! This is what causes the inflammation or tendonitis, and whether the sport is running, football, basketball, track, or even golf, the proper shoe can help prevent painful problems.

Metatarsalgia

Another injury we encounter regularly is metatarsalgia. It's a common condition in which the ball of the foot becomes painful and inflamed. Activities that involve running and jumping are frequently the cause. The great news is that proper footwear can alleviate symptoms and prevent future problems. Often, treatment will include placing a pad beneath the metatarsal to relieve pressure from the ball of the foot. This allows for shock absorption through a better insole in the shoe.

Essentially, this pad gives a little more cushion to the ball of the foot. Our goal is to off-load (decrease) as much pressure from the metatarsal as possible.

Some of the pads we use are common items you can buy in a store, but it's still wise to drop by so we can ensure it is properly placed. Pressure needs to be alleviated from the right places and we have the expertise to ensure that happens. For instance, with runners, we usually see the issue on the inside leg of the track. This happens because when they run laps around the track, the inside leg endures more pressure. So when you come in, we focus precisely on what is causing your pain or injury, and then treat accordingly.

Patella Femoral Syndrome

As a pedorthist, when I see a runner with knee pain, I can almost always fix it through the foot. In most cases, we simply need to get the knee in alignment with the foot and the ankle for a smoother motion. When the knee is out of alignment with the foot and ankle, patella femoral syndrome can result, which is a misalignment between the patella (kneecap) and the knee joint that causes pain.

The patella is designed to glide over the knee joint as it extends. However, due to hyper-pronation of the foot (flat foot), it migrates and rubs against the condyles of the femur. This pressure is where the pain comes from. The cartilage under your kneecap is a natural shock absorber and is meant to help prevent issues like these, but with overuse, injury, or misalignments, this condition can occur. The most common symptom is knee pain that increases when you walk up or down stairs.

Simple treatments like rest and ice can help, but sometimes physical therapy and custom-built orthotics are needed to relieve the patellofemoral pain. When we fit inserts to correct this issue, we generally use rigid orthotics that include both hind-foot and fore-foot posting to keep the ankle in a neutral position. Both of these help to relieve pressure from the knee and take away pain beneath the patella.

Medial Tibial Stress Syndrome

Though you've likely heard it by its simpler name, shin splints, medial tibial stress syndrome is perhaps the most common sports-related injury we treat. Shin splints are a pain along the large bone in the shin called the tibia. Shin splints result from hyperpronation through the gait cycle, improper shock absorption, weakness in the posterior tibial muscle, or overtraining. The muscle pulls the foot into position for toe-off which causes stress on the inside of the shin.

To fix this, we need to get the foot into a neutral position and relieve the problematic stress. Our primary means of doing this is through orthotics. What is important to remember is that athletes are vulnerable to foot injuries because of their sport's specific mechanical requirements, so if we build an orthotic that supports them in their sport, it can provide an edge and prevention of injuries. Again, injuries are the last thing we want because our athletes are out of the game and unable to participate. To properly fit athletes, both podiatrists and pedorthists need to understand the mechanics of the sport, and the mentality of the athlete, to align to the prescribed treatment.

The Right Shoe For Your Sport

Have you ever considered shoes to be a part of your sports equipment? Well, they are. They're your first point of contact with the playing surface and are a part of who you are when you're engaged in a sport. Shoes also have a significant impact on performance. We have pads and helmets for football so we can smash into people without being hurt, but do we have the right cleat for our feet? Tennis players may have the right racket, but what about a shoe that supports their quick sprints and leaps? The same goes for golfers and track athletes. To prevent injuries we need the proper footwear designed for our sport.

In addition to injury prevention, being in the right shoe or orthotic can help the athlete perform at the top of his or her game. Should a boxer use gloves that are heavier than necessary? Should a catcher use an ill-fitting mitt? Or a soccer player use shin guards that only protect halfway up the shin? Obviously not! We know that performance is hampered when we don't have the right equipment. Our feet are no different. They need the proper footwear to do their job well and give them the edge of peak performance.

We know that the right shoes and orthotics are important to performance, but how do we know which shoe will work best? There are four primary questions we ask to discern this. First, what is the duration of the athlete's training time? What is the practice frequency? Are practices held a few times during the week, or will it be two-a-days? Is he or she a distance runner? If yes, then how many miles a week will be put on the shoes? We need to understand everything the shoe will need to do for the athlete—especially outside of game day.

Next, we consider the intensity of performance. A golfer needs a much different shoe than a basketball player for many obvious reasons. One reason is a difference in intensity. We want to know how intense the athlete's activities are going to be and will select a shoe that can properly support them.

Another reason why a golfer and a basketball player require a very different shoe is because of the playing surfaces. A hardwood court is much different than manicured Bermuda grass. Likewise, a marathoner pounding out miles on the pavement will need a much different shoe than a football player on the turf.

And lastly, we also take into account the athlete's physical history: weight, foot type, foot size, foot shape, and current and previous injuries. Is the individual's foot wide or narrow? Does he or she have a high arch or flat foot? Are there any current injuries that need to be treated or past injuries that need to be prevented from recurring? A credentialed pedorthist will be able to take these factors into consideration and find the shoe that provides the proper cushion, support, and protection.

Most sports require the foot to perform concurrent and opposing movements. Start and stop. Forwards and backwards. Side to side. All too often, if you're in the wrong shoe, we'll see things like metatarsal fractures and achilles tendonitis occur because of these demands. Think of it like this: you're not going to put a pair of thirty-five inch mud-flapper tires on your car or truck to go cruising down the interstate. Why? Because they're not going to perform the way you want and need them to. The same principal applies for athletes. You've got to make sure you're wearing the right shoe for your sport.

The Right Orthotic For Your Sport

Just like shoe selection, we build orthotics specifically for your sports based on the sports specific mechanics. Again, we won't make the same orthotic for a golfer and a basketball player. Most of the time a golfer walks in a straight line while a basketball player is cutting and weaving, jumping high, and landing hard.

A basketball player will need something with shock absorption and a softer heel. The basketball player needs something that takes the sheer force applied to the ball of the foot because they're pivoting and turning. Their forefoot also needs support as their gait will see a lot of lateral motion. Similar to the shoes, our process also takes into account playing surfaces and the impact they'll have on the athlete's joints and ligaments. We design and build the orthotic with the athlete's surface needs in mind. Ultimately, when we get them properly fit, the athlete is going to be able to perform at a higher level with fewer injuries.

Whether it is baseball season in the spring or football season in the fall, Fit My Feet should be your first stop. We'll consider an athlete's diagnosis and how it can be corrected. We'll take a look at the unique physical demands of the sports he or she plays and fit according to the mechanical and playing surface. In the end, these are the details that inform the kind of shoe we fit them in and the kind of orthotic that we build for them.

Question 1

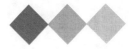

Do I wear the proper shoe for the sport I play?

Question 2

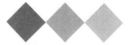

When was the last time I had my feet measured in order to find the right shoe?

Question 3

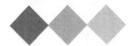

Have I had a recurring injury that may be addressed with a different shoe or orthotic?

Biography

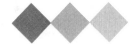

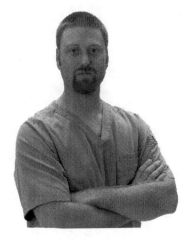

Nick Kolterman

www.FitMyFeet.biz
FMFOAS@gmail.com
605-274-0138
2105 S Minnesota Ave
Sioux Falls, SD 57105

Thank you for reading my book. In addition to being a board certified pedorthist, I have a very strong passion in what I do helping patients. I have spent years studying gait analysis to put people into the right shoes and orthotics. I have also been to many seminars and lectures over the years to better my education in helping people live a pain-free life. I work with a knowledgeable group of physicians within our community to get their patients back to health. It is our job to work in reference with the physician or other licensed healthcare prescriber including MD, DC, DPM, PT and DO to help fabricate the correct orthotic, shoe or brace to help with feet, hip, back or knee problems. We evaluate all aspects of biomechanics.

As a Pedorthist, we are the EXPERTS who design, manufacture, modify and fit footwear, including custom foot and ankle orthoses, to alleviate foot problems caused by disease, overuse, or injury.

My care toward the patient is treating you like I would treat one of my family. I look forward to helping you get back to health.